# Clean Eating

### Lean Diet Plans to Help Lose Weight, Gain Energy and Be Happy & Healthy

I0423425

## L.T. Currow

Copyright © 2016 L.T. Currow

ISBN:
ISBN-13: 978-1533515377

ISBN-10: 1533515379

# CONTENTS

# INTRODUCTION

Congratulations on downloading *Clean Eating: Lean Diet Plans to Help Lose Weight, Gain Energy and Be Happy and Healthy.*

In this book, you will find a number of diet plans that will help you get rid of unwanted weight and fat while boosting your energy simultaneously, all through the practice of clean eating.

Regardless of your experience with diets or calorie counting in the past, in the chapters ahead, you will find a plan that will leave you feeling better about yourself, physically and mentally, than you did when you first opened this book. Happiness and health are two things that we all strive for in life and one of the best ways to achieve both of those goals is by feeding your body in the best way possible. By reading ahead, you will find out how to do just that.

Thank you for reading *Clean Eating*, enjoy every minute of it. Stay happy and stay healthy!

# 1 THE DANGERS OF UNHEALTHY EATING

As human beings who belong and function in a society, we may or may not be aware that our eating patterns and food choices are largely dictated by the world we live in. For example, population studies show that there are stark differences between the food and nutrient intake among social classes, with low-income groups having a greater tendency to consume unbalanced diets, which are energy-rich yet nutrient poor, and low on fruit and vegetables. Meanwhile, those who belong to high-income groups have a tendency to consume too much food items that are laden with unhealthy fat.[1] These unhealthy diets not only affect our body, but they can likewise cause behavioral health issues, and affect how a person feels, looks, thinks and acts, resulting in lower body core strength, slower problem-solving ability and muscle

---

[1] What we eat what we eat: Social and Economic Determinants of Food Choice. European Food Information Council. Can be accessed at http://www.eufic.org/article/en/ health-and-lifestyle/food-choice/artid/social-economic-determinants-food-choice/. Last accessed on 4 April 2016.

response time, and less alertness. Unhealthy eating has its dangers, and if left unmitigated, will result in several severe health problems, such as the following:

## Obesity

In a study by the World Health Organization, it was stated that the worldwide obesity rate has more than doubled since 1980. Moreover, in 2014, there are at least 1.9 billion adults who are deemed overweight, 600 Million of whom were classified as obese. This rise in the global incidence of obesity can be largely attributed to two key factors: (1) an increase in the intake of calorie-dense food items; and (2) a significant lack of physical activity due to modern lifestyle including the sedentary nature of many jobs, as well as developments in technology that contributed to such a lifestyle.

As a person's body mass index rises, the risk of developing Coronary Heart Disease also rises. Coronary Heart Disease is a condition in which plaque, a waxy substance, accumulates inside the coronary arteries and blocks the supply of oxygen-rich blood to the heart, which eventually leads to a heart attack. Obesity is also a risk factor in heart failure, as the heart is no longer able to pump blood due to the more taxing demands of an obese body.[2]

Aside from heart issues, an overweight or obese person has an increased risk of getting a stroke, which results from the buildup of plaque in the arteries in the

---

[2] What are the Health Risks of Overweight and Obesity? National Heart, Ling, and Blood Institute. Can be accessed at https://www.nhlbi.nih.gov/health/health-topics/topics/obe/risks. Last accessed on 4 April 2016.

brain. The area with the build-up will eventually rupture, causing blood clot to form.[3]

An overweight or obese person can also develop Type 2 Diabetes due to the high sugar in the blood. Normally, our body will produce insulin to turn the excess glucose into energy. However, the continuous consumption of foods rich in sugar will trigger our body to continuously produce insulin until such time that it can no longer keep up with our body's demands, leaving the sugar level in the blood uncontrolled.[4]

### Metabolic Problems

The consumption of unhealthy foods can also affect a person's metabolic functions. Consumption of junk foods and other processed foods for five (5) days disrupts our body's ability to oxidize glucose. According to the study, the normal response to a meal was blunted or absent after five (5) days of high-fat feeding. However, when normal food was consumed, there was big increases in oxidative targets within four (4) hours after the meal. The delay in the oxidization process can lead to inflammation problems, constriction of blood vessels, elevated free radicals levels, rise in blood pressure. Moreover, the surge and drop in insulin brought about by the glucose concentration in the blood will make an

---

[3] What are the Health Risks of Overweight and Obesity? National Heart, Ling, and Blood Institute. Can be accessed at https://www.nhlbi.nih.gov/health/health-topics/topics/obe/risks. Last accessed on 4 April 2016.

[4] What are the Health Risks of Overweight and Obesity? National Heart, Ling, and Blood Institute. Can be accessed at https://www.nhlbi.nih.gov/health/health-topics/topics/obe/risks. Last accessed on 4 April 2016.

individual crave food more frequently even though his body is not in need of extra energy. [5]

Worse, fathers who consume junk food may pass metabolic disorders to their children. A research conducted on mice found that unhealthy eating behaviors were recorded in a tiny molecule that could be transmitted through the sperm to the embryo. If this happens, the offspring of a parent who became obese through a diet of junk food can become inclined to consume substantial levels of glucose.[6]

Cancer

Research has shown that poor diet and inactivity are two (2) key factors that can increase a person's risk of developing cancer. As a matter of fact, the World Cancer Research Fund approximates that about twenty percent (20%) of all diagnosed cancers in the United States are related to weight gain, physical inactivity, excessive alcohol intake, and poor nutrition. Moreover, studies have linked eating red or processed meat to an increased risk of breast cancer, colon cancer, prostate cancer, and pancreatic cancer, which may be caused by carcinogens in food which were cooked in high temperatures.

Bone Diseases

---

[5] What Happens to Your Body When You Eat Junk Food? Can be accessed at http://articles.mercola.com/sites/articles/archive/2015/04/29/junk-food-metabolism.aspx. Last accessed on 4 April 2016.

[6] Junk Food Eating Generations Can Pass Metabolic Disorders to Their Children. Can be accessed at http://preventdisease.com/news/16/011316_Junk-Food-Eating-Generations-Pass-Metabolic-Disorders-Children.shtml. Last accessed on 4 April 2016.

Malnutrition can also affect the body's bones and cause long-term diseases such as osteoarthritis wherein the tissue that protects our joints wears away. As we age, our bones regenerate at a slower pace. As a result, we lose more bone density than what our bodies can regenerate. If we do not support our bone regeneration through a healthy intake of food, our bones can become brittle over time.

### Lethargy

Eating too much food too quickly will cause a person to feel heavy and tired because our body re-directs a large volume of our blood from our head to our digestive system, resulting in lowered blood pressure and dizziness. Moreover, a study published in Physiology & Behavior observes that rats which were fed with junk food shows impaired performance on simple tasks as compared to other rats which were fed with normal food. In said tests, the junk-food fed rats took breaks which were twice as long as the other rats.[7] Another study suggests that children with unhealthy eating habits, especially those whose diets are rich in salty foods, feel more tired throughout the day.[8]

As the old adage says, we are what we eat. However, we often indulge in eating as a coping mechanism or a social function that we forget that the

---

[7] Does A Junk Food Diet Make You Lazy and Fatigued? Regularly Eating Processed Foods Linked to Cognitive Impairment. Can be Accessed at http:// www.medicaldaily.com/does-junk-food-diet-make-you-lazy-and-fatigued-regularly-eating-processed-foods-linked-cognitive. Last Accessed on 4 April 2016.

[8] Are you Tired All the Time? Food Might be to Blame. Can be accessed at: http://psychcentral.com/blog/archives/2012/10/16/are-you-tired-all-the-time-food-might-be-to-blame/ Last accessed on 4 April 2016.

primary role of food is to fuel or body's daily needs. Unfortunately, though we have the freedom to choose what to set on the table, we cannot choose the consequences of our poor eating habits. However, it is not too late to change, and we can all change our eating habits for the better.

# 2 PRELUDE TO HEALTHY EATING - DETOXIFY!

The consumption of junk food and other processed food can leave a lot of toxins and free radicals in our body that could create problems and induce cravings once we start eating clean and healthy food. For example, a person who is used to foods with high sugar content will feel light headed and nauseous during the first days of his diet plan, and may cause him to revert to his usual high-sugar diet. So in order to properly prepare the body to clean eating, it is advisable that a person detoxify his body first.

The fastest, but albeit the hardest, way to detoxify the body is through water fasting. During water fasting, the individual can only drink water for a day or several days in order to flush out toxins and free radicals in the body. It also aids in cleansing organs that helps detoxify the liver, kidneys, lungs, and lymphatics, to name a few. Keep this seven (7) tips in mind during your fast:

1.  Consult a doctor - Before undergoing a fast, be sure to ask your physician first if it is advisable for you to fast, as there are specific conditions that are

counter-indicative for fasting such as pregnancy, immune disorders, eating disorders, and chronic ailments such as heart disease. The prescription of specific medications can also make it unsafe for some patients to undergo a fast.

2. Plan - Fasting, or even just the thought of it, can be taxing mentally. Hence, a plan will help you to commit to the fast. Also, you have to schedule the fast in such a way that your daily activities would not interfere with it. It will be best if you will be able to rest during your entire fast.

3. Eat only vegetables and fruits prior to fast- Before the fast, eat only plant-based food with no oil, sugar, or salt several days before the fast. This will prevent dizziness, nausea, headaches, and food "withdrawals" during the first few days of the fast and improve the over-all experience.

4. Anticipate discomfort – If it is your first time to fast, and you were accustomed to poor lifestyle, expect certain discomforts during the first few days of the fast as your body adjust to the lack of food and the excretion of toxins from your body. In certain cases, drugs and toxic chemicals that are in your system get flushed out during the fast. You will start to feel better once these toxic chemicals are out of your body.

5. Drink enough water- It is recommended that you get anywhere between 8 to 10 8oz glasses of water per day in the fast, more depending on weather and physical activity. It is advisable if you drink

distilled water only, since this type of water is pure $H_2O$, and free from inorganic minerals which will harm your body. Health problems caused by these inorganic minerals include kidney stones, gallbladder, and the development of stone-like acid crystals in the person's veins, arteries, and other body parts. In case the fasting occurred during hot weather, the water intake should be increased to compensate for water-loss due to sweating.

6. Get enough rest- While rest is important no matter what you are doing, getting enough rest must be emphasized during water fasting. As mentioned earlier, fasting is a physically taxing experience. There would be a lot of times where you'll feel very tired. A drop in stamina and overall energy would be experienced, especially during the first three (3) days of fasting. This is because your body is adjusting to the absence of food, switching to your internal energy reserves, and busy expelling all your toxins out. Don't overexert yourself during this fasting period and make sure to get enough sleep.

7. Avoid high-intensity exercise- Remember that during a fast, your energy levels might be on an all-time low. There are other low-intensity exercises you can try to maintain in shape while putting minimal strain on your body. One example of such exercise is yoga. It ensures muscle strength and flexibility are not compromised. It can also aid in the detoxification process. You're free to exercise during fasting, as long as you keep the intensity to manageable levels.

If water fasting is too much, an individual may resort to juice cleansing. Juice cleansing is a fasting method or a detoxification diet in which a person only consumes blended fruits and vegetable to obtain nutrition while abstaining from solid foods. Proponents of juice cleansing encourages practitioners to consume blends made from eighty percent (80%) vegetables and twenty percent (20%) fruits, in order to avoid excess sugar in the blend, while maintaining high nutrient value. Be sure, however, to use fruits and vegetables that are fibrous during the juice cleansing process and include the pulp of the vegetables and fruit in the blend, as participants may have trouble relieving their bowels due to the lack of fiber content of the blends they consume.

Following are some juice cleansing recipes:

Juice #1:

- 2 Apples, medium size
- 1 Cucumber, medium
- 4 Celery stalks
- Ginger Root,1 thumb
- 6 leaves of Kale
- ½ Lemon

Directions: Mix all the ingredients in the blender.


The combination of the ingredients can: (1) aid in weight loss; (2) improve complexion; (3) lower blood pressure; (4) prevent cataracts, colon cancer, breast cancer, liver cancer, lung cancer, Alzheimer's, osteoporosis, asthma, heart disease, and inflammation; (5) improve the immune system; (6) aid the digestion; and (7) increase blood circulation.

Juice #2:

- 1 Apple, medium, cored and peeled
- 4 Carrots, medium, peeled
- ¼ Lemon
- 8 fl. Oz of Green Tea
- A teaspoon of honey.
- 1 peeled Orange - deseeded

Directions:

1. Make a separate cup of green tea. Steep the green tea in hot water for three (3) minutes. Add honey to this mixture.

2. Process all the other ingredients in the juicer.

3. Pour green tea mixture into the juice. Pulse until mixed thoroughly. Serve.

This specific juice is great for: (1) digestion; (2) improved complexion; (3) immune system; (4) lowered cholesterol; (5) lung cancer prevention; (6) heart disease prevention; (7) improving eyesight; (8) macular degeneration prevention; (9) reduced water retention; (10) stroke prevention; (11) cancer prevention; (12) stomach cancer prevention; (13) asthma help; (14) breast cancer prevention; (15) Alzheimer's prevention; (16) bone protection; (17) colon cancer prevention; (18) liver cancer prevention; (19) lowered blood pressure; and (20) weight loss.

Juice #3:

- 8 carrots, medium

- 2 stalks of Celery
- 1 apple, medium
- 1 Beet Root
- 3 cups of spinach

Directions: Mix all the ingredients in the blender.

# 3 TO EAT OR NOT TO EAT

A lot of diet fads today focus too much on the calorie intake and portion control without taking into consideration satiety and the body's nutrient intake. Thus, the end results usually falls short of the outcome. Sure, an individual may lose weight, but since the diet is not sustainable, the person will just return to his or her prior lifestyle, causing his or her to regain the lost weight. What is needed to teach individuals to eat clean healthy food which will be able to supply the body with the nutrients in needs, promotes satiety, and eliminates unhealthy cravings. Once a person develops this lifestyle, weight loss is sure to follow.

The journey to clean eating starts with consciously avoiding foods that are harmful to your body and sticking to whole foods. Whole foods are the kind of food that is unprocessed and unrefined. These are foods derived from nature, be that a farm, a garden, a field, or an orchard, that have not been to artificially produced insecticides and grown in soil fertilized only by biological wastes and composts.

Examples of whole foods are unpolished grains and beans, as well as fruits, vegetables, meats, and non-homogenized dairy products. Processed foods, on the other hand, may be convenient and tasty, but are high in chemical additives, trans-fat, salt, and sugar. Processed foods are, more or less, already pre-digested due to the procedure which they go through. Hence, it takes our body less time to digest them, leading to a spike in the sugar levels in our blood. Moreover, a lot of the nutrients in the food are eliminated because of the method by which food companies process these food items. Thus, our aim is to stock on unprocessed foods that can supply our body with the most nutrients, keep the blood sugar level even, and can produce sustained release of energy for our body. Thus, during grocery shopping, keep these sixteen (16) tips in mind to guide you on what to put in your shopping cart:

1. Avoid foods and goods that came in boxes or packaging. Usually, processed foods are re-packed and labeled to pro-long shelf life. Of course, there are a few exceptions to the rule, such as packed greens, however, most packaged goods such as flour, noodles, sauces, hotdogs, hams, canned goods and the like, are usually already refined and loaded with chemicals and preservatives to enhance flavor and pro-long shelf life. Moreover, canned goods are often lined with aluminum and plastic membrane which contain a chemicals which may be harmful for you.


2. Choose brown or black rice over white rice. The color of unpolished rice is brown or black. Brown or black rice has more fiber, protein, and nutrients such as proteins, thiamine, calcium, magnesium, fiber, and potassium, than white rice. Brown rice also makes you feel fuller, and takes longer time to digest than white rice. Meanwhile,

white polished rice is energy-rich, but lacks nutrients. Hence, it floods your system with sugar, but it does not give your body the nutrients that it needs. Other types of unpolished grains include millet, amaranth, and quinoa.

3.   Look for clean sugar substitutes such as honey, maple syrup, and dehydrated sugar cane juice. If you don't feel like using sugar substitute, avoid washed sugar and buy brown sugar instead. The darker the color of the sugar, the better. Also, avoid commercially produced honey as producers usually add sugar to it. You may source your honey from a local bee keeper.

4.   Avoid canned or artificial juices. Buy whole fruits and vegetables and juice them instead. Packed fruit juices are usually loaded with preservatives. It is better to be sure that what you drink is fresh.

5.   It goes without saying that soda should be off your list. Sodas are loaded with sugar which will cause your blood sugar to spike. In response, your body will produce large amounts of insulin to normalize your blood sugar level, leaving you shaky, weak, and more hungry.

6.   Avoid smoked or processed meats and fish, because it is possible that additives and preservatives were already included in the product to pro-long shelf live and prevent the

discoloration of the meat. You may opt to buy fresh meats and fish and smoke them yourself, or choose to buy from smaller producers instead.

7.      Be careful when buying processed vegetarian food such as quorn and soy meat replacements. These are heavily processed and loaded with additives. Be sure to inspect the label properly when buying. You may also opt to purchase from smaller producers.

8.      Avoid buying pre-made seasonings. A lot of the handy, prepared seasoning products are already preserved with sulphur dioxide. Instead, prepare your own seasoning. You may buy fresh garlic, ginger, or chili, and prepare the seasoning yourself. You may chill or freeze your prepared seasonings. When buying flavoring like vanilla extract, make sure to check the labels to find out if the product contains ethanol and additional sugar.    To avoid these chemicals, you may use seeds from a vanilla pod.

9.      Avoid condiments and dressings. Condiments such as mayonnaise, ketchup, salad dressings, and mustard contain additives like sugar. They may also contain poor quality or unhealthy vegetable oil. Instead, you may opt to use other alternatives to these condiments. For example, instead of using ketchup, you may prepare and use fresh tomato salsa. Also, instead of using heavy salad dressing, opt to prepare and use vinaigrettes

instead, using olive oil, apple cider vinegar, and your choice of herbs.

10. Refrain from buying dried fruits as these are already loaded with sweeteners and other chemicals such as sulphur dioxide. If you must buy dried fruit, look for those which were sweetened naturally using honey or apple juice.

11. Refrain from buying margarines. Aside from artificial colorings, additives, and emulsifiers to improve appearance, margarines contains chemically hardened vegetable oil. Also, margarines contains trans fat, a type of fat which is not recognized by the body, and hence, may contribute to heart diseases, cancer, bone problems, hormonal imbalance, skin disease, and other health issues. It is better to just use clarified butter, or ghee, than margarine. Clarified butter is butter that has been melted over low hear and allowed to bubble and simmer until most of the water has been evaporated. Butter, despite common misconception about its health benefits, consists of butterfat, as well as some milk proteins. Butterfat is also known as butyric acid -- the same substance found in a mother's milk. Other beneficial components of butter include:

    a. anti-oxidants such as beta-carotene, selenium, that shield your body from free-radical damage;

b. conjugated linoleic acids, which fights cancer, builds muscle, and boost immunity;

c. iodine, which keeps the thyroid glands healthy;

d. lauric acid, which boosts the immune system and makes it better at fighting infections;

e. lecithin, which has powerful antioxidant properties, and also contributes to cholesterol metabolism, and

f. vitamins A, D, E, and K, which are essential for eye and endocrine health, calcium absorption, healing, skin health, and proper blood clotting.

12. Choose high quality meat. Aim to get your meat from grass-fed animals as much as possible. It may be more expensive, but it is a lot healthier than animals which were fed with feeds which were also loaded with chemicals from factories. If you have space and ability, you may also raise your own chickens. If there is no option but to purchase lower quality meat, go for the leaner cuts, as chemicals can accumulate in the fatty tissues.

13. Include Healthy Fats. Our body needs fats, so do not be afraid to consume healthy, high-quality saturated fats. Healthy fats is found in fish,

such as white tuna, salmon, anchovies and sardines; nuts and seeds such as walnuts, almonds, pecans, chia, flax and hemp seeds; avocados; eggs; and oils such as real butter, olive oil and virgin coconut oil.

14. Consume as many vegetables as you can during your meals. Opt for cruciferous, dark leafy greens. The idea, however, is to have variety of vegetables as possible in your diet, the more colorful, the better.

15. Limit your drink to water. If you must, stick to green tea, coconut water, and aloe vera juice. Moderate the intake of coffee.

16. For purposes of weight loss, you may want to stock up on these foods:

    a. Whole eggs. Eggs are high in protein, healthy fats, and can make you feel full with a very low amount of calories. In a study of overweight women, it was showed that eating eggs for breakfast increased satiety and caused the women to eat less for the next thirty-six (36) hours.

    b. Leafy greens and cruciferous vegetables. Leafy greens and cruciferous vegetables are loaded with fiber while containing low carbohydrates. Eating leafy greens and cruciferous vegetables during meals can help you consume less calories while getting enough nutrients and satiety. The fiber in the food will also help regulate bowel movement. Cruciferous vegetables includes broccoli, cauliflower, cabbage, garden cress, and brussels sprouts.

c. Seafood. Seafood contains iodine, which is necessary for the proper function of the thyroid, which regulates metabolism.

d. Lean Beef and Chicken Breast. Unprocessed lean beef and chicken breast contains a lot of protein, which is the most fulfilling nutrient. Eating a high-protein diet can make you burn up to a hundred more calories per day.

e. Beans and Legumes. Beans and legumes are high in protein and fiber, which will help a person feel full. Beans and legumes also contain resistant starch, which allows for sustained energy release.

f. Cottage Cheese. Cheese in general is high in protein. However, cottage cheese has the highest amount of protein, and very little carbohydrate and fat.

g. Avocados. Avocados are loaded with healthy fats and high in monounsaturated oleic acid, which is the same fat found in olive oil. Avocados are perfect additions to salads, as studies have shown that fats in avocados increases the nutrient uptake from the vegetables.

h. Apple Cider Vinegar (ACV). Taking ACV at the same time as a high carbohydrate meal can increase the feeling of fullness and can make a person eat less calories throughout the day. ACV can also aid digestion and regulate bowel movement.

i. Grapefruit. Studies have shown that people who eat grapefruit before meals where able to lose weight. Moreover, grapefruit can help people suffering from insulin resistance and metabolic abnormality.

j.   Chia Seeds. Chia seeds is one of the best source of fiber known to man. Because of its fiber content, these seeds can absorb up to 11-12 times of their weight in water, expands in the stomach, and makes a person feel full.

You may try this five (5) day meal plan which applies the above principles to get you started!

Day 1:

| Breakfast - Wholegrain cereal with milk, topped with ½ cup blue berries and 200 g. low fat fruit yogurt. |
| --- |
| Lunch – Tuna salad roll<br><br>You will need:<br><br>1 Wholemeal roll, sliced avocadoes, chopped tune (cooked), cheese, carrot strips, 2 slices of beetroot, and cucumber slices. |

Dinner- Baked lean turkey breast with vegetables

You will need:

200g Turkey breast, glazed in honey or marinated in sauce, steamed squash and broccoli as sides.

Snacks - Whole-wheat bread topped with cottage cheese and fresh tomato, green tea.

Day 2:

Breakfast – 1 toasted whole meal flat bread topped with cheese. 1 banana and 20g wholegrain cereal with skimmed milk.

Lunch – Wholemeal beef bread roll

You will need:

1 wholemeal, 60g Lean roast beef, avocado slices, 2 tsp honey, grated carrots, chopped cucumber, and lettuce

## Dinner

Marinated chicken skewers and chickpea salad

You will need:

200 g Chicken breast marinated in 1 tsp olive oil, cumin, fresh garlic, coriander, and mint

¾ cup Chick pea, ½ cup English spinach, ¼ cup cherry tomatoes, 3 onion rings, 1 tsb parsley, and citrus dressing,

## Snacks

1 apple, diced and mixed with low-fat yogurt, green tea.

Day 3:

Breakfast – Mixed fruits (we recommend: apples, pears, bananas, and oranges – or any combination thereof) topped with about 200g of vanilla yogurt and 20g whole grain cereal.

Lunch – Wholemeal tuna bread roll

You will need:

1 wholemeal, 60g tuna, 2 tsp honey, grated carrots, chopped cucumber, tettuce

Dinner

Vegetable soup and garlic prawns

You will need:

Cauliflower, beans, broccoli, carrots

Sauteed garlic and prawns

1 heavily seeded bread roll and butter

Snacks

Two soy linseed corn crispbreads and green tea. Optional: top bread with cheese.

Day 4:

| |
|---|
| Breakfast – 40g cereal, wholegrain, topped with 200g vanilla yogurt, a tablespoon of chia seeds, 3 prunes and 3 apricot halves (dried) |
| Lunch – Crispbread topped with eggs and tuna<br><br>You will need:<br><br>4 crispbread, egg, tuna<br><br>1 apple |
| Dinner<br><br>Creamy chicken pasta<br><br>You will need:<br><br>200g skinless chicken breast, ¼ cup light evaporated milk, chicken stock, 4 asparagus spears, ¼ cup frozen peas and corn, 1 cup cooked wholemeal pasta |
| Snacks<br><br>Fruit slices of your choice |

Day 5:

Breakfast – apple and banana smoothie, with 40g wholegrain cereal with skim milk

Lunch – Sardines on toast

You will need:

2 slices wholemeal toast, butter, and sardines in tomato sauce

1 cup of green grapes

Dinner

Beef and spinach pasta and salad

You will need:

200g lean beef, ½ cup English spinach, ¼ cup light evaporated milk, tomato puree, fress garlic and basil, 1 cup cooked wholemeal pasta

½ cup lettuce, ¼ cup mushrooms, sliced cucumber, 5 olives, 1 tsp olive oil, ½ tsp balsamic vinegar, and ½ tsp honey, wholegrain mustard

Snacks

Mixed apple, banana, and orange, topped with light cream.

Keep in mind that the following are mere guidelines to help you in achieving a healthier lifestyle, as there is no one-size-fits-all definition of clean eating. The general rule is to eat wholesome foods, and avoid chemically laden food. Keep in mind that each individual has a different genetic make-up, and hence, our dietary needs are different. Also clean eating is not merely a phase, or a diet that you can do for a week, or a month, in order for you to lose weight. Your decision to live healthy and eat clean, wholesome foods must be a lifestyle change, which ultimately redefines your relationship with food. Otherwise, the exercise will be futile.

Moreover, keep in mind that clean eating is not equivalent to self-deprivation. Sure, you may be taking in fewer calories than before, but it does not mean that you will starve yourself. As a matter of fact, eating clean can allow you to eat more. You might be surprise to know that a quarter bar of your favorite white chocolate has the same calorie content as a big bowl of greens! Also, eating lean proteins such as chicken breast, fish, tofu, and green such as broccoli, kale, lettuce, green beans, together with whole grains like quinoa, oatmeal, and brown rice can keep you feel fuller for a longer time.

Keep in mind also that the goal of clean eating is not to frustrate the individual, but to keep him or her happy and healthy. Hence, if you really want to try that piece of cake in a party, do it, but do not over do it. The idea is to live healthy most of the time, not to have a perfect tract record.

# 4 HEALTHY PORTIONS: JUST HOW MUCH IS ENOUGH?

It is not enough that you know what you should and what you should not eat. It is also important to know just how many you should eat. Too little food intake can be as damaging as too much food intake. Starving yourself can lead to muscle loss, decreased energy, malnutrition, and lowered metabolic functions. On the other hand, eating too much, even though they are the right food, can nullify your efforts to lose weight, and live a healthy lifestyle.

Our problem with portion control is further exacerbated by the increases in food servings at commercial areas as a way to compete in the market. Hence, what seems like a normal serving size a decade ago seem small in comparison today. As a matter of A lot of diet fads today focus too much on the calorie intake and portion control without taking into consideration satiety and the body's nutrient intake. Thus, the end results usually falls short of the outcome. Sure, an individual may lose weight, but since the diet is not sustainable, the person will just return to his or her prior lifestyle, causing his or her to regain the lost weight. What is needed to teach individuals to eat clean healthy food which will be able to supply the body with the nutrients in needs, promotes satiety, and eliminates unhealthy cravings. Once a person develops this lifestyle, weight loss is sure to follow.

The journey to clean eating starts with consciously avoiding foods that are harmful to your body and sticking to whole foods. Whole foods are the kind of food that is unprocessed and unrefined. These are foods derived from nature, be that a farm, a garden, a field, or an orchard, that have not been to artificially produced insecticides and grown in soil fertilized only by biological wastes and composts.

Examples of whole foods are unpolished grains and beans, as well as fruits, vegetables, meats, and non-homogenized dairy products. Processed foods, on the other hand, may be convenient and tasty, but are high in chemical additives, trans-fat, salt, and sugar. Processed foods are, more or less, already pre-digested due to the procedure which they go through. Hence, it takes our body less time to digest them, leading to a spike in the sugar levels in our blood. Moreover, a lot of the nutrients in the food are eliminated because of the method by which food companies process these food items. Thus, our aim is to stock on unprocessed foods that can supply our body with the most nutrients, keep the blood sugar level even, and can produce sustained release of energy for our body. Thus, during grocery shopping, keep these sixteen (16) tips in mind to guide you on what to put in your shopping cart:

    1.   Avoid foods and goods that came in boxes or packaging. Usually, processed foods are re-packed and labeled to pro-long shelf life. Of course, there are a few exceptions to the rule, such as packed greens, however, most packaged goods such as flour, noodles, sauces, hotdogs, hams, canned goods and the like, are usually already refined and loaded with chemicals and preservatives to enhance flavor and pro-long shelf

life. Moreover, canned goods are often lined with aluminum and plastic membrane which contain a chemicals which may be harmful for you.

2. Choose brown or black rice over white rice. The color of unpolished rice is brown or black. Brown or black rice has more fiber, protein, and nutrients such as proteins, thiamine, calcium, magnesium, fiber, and potassium, than white rice. Brown rice also makes you feel fuller, and takes longer time to digest than white rice. Meanwhile, white polished rice is energy-rich, but lacks nutrients. Hence, it floods your system with sugar, but it does not give your body the nutrients that it needs. Other types of unpolished grains include millet, amaranth, and quinoa.

3. Look for clean sugar substitutes such as honey, maple syrup, and dehydrated sugar cane juice. If you don't feel like using sugar substitute, avoid washed sugar and buy brown sugar instead. The darker the color of the sugar, the better. Also, avoid commercially produced honey as producers usually add sugar to it. You may source your honey from a local bee keeper.

4. Avoid canned or artificial juices. Buy whole fruits and vegetables and juice them instead. Packed fruit juices are usually loaded with preservatives. It is better to be sure that what you drink is fresh.

5.    It goes without saying that soda should be off your list. Sodas are loaded with sugar which will cause your blood sugar to spike. In response, your body will produce large amounts of insulin to normalize your blood sugar level, leaving you shaky, weak, and more hungry.

6.    Avoid smoked or processed meats and fish, because it is possible that additives and preservatives were already included in the product to pro-long shelf live and prevent the discoloration of the meat. You may opt to buy fresh meats and fish and smoke them yourself, or choose to buy from smaller producers instead.

7.    Be careful when buying processed vegetarian food such as quorn and soy meat replacements. These are heavily processed and loaded with additives. Be sure to inspect the label properly when buying. You may also opt to purchase from smaller producers.

8.    Avoid buying pre-made seasonings. A lot of the handy, prepared seasoning products are already preserved with sulphur dioxide. Instead, prepare your own seasoning. You may buy fresh garlic, ginger, or chili, and prepare the seasoning yourself. You may chill or freeze your prepared seasonings. When buying flavoring like vanilla extract, make sure to check the labels to find out if the product contains ethanol and additional sugar.    To avoid these chemicals, you may use seeds from a vanilla pod.

9.  Avoid condiments and dressings. Condiments such as mayonnaise, ketchup, salad dressings, and mustard contain additives like sugar. They may also contain poor quality or unhealthy vegetable oil. Instead, you may opt to use other alternatives to these condiments. For example, instead of using ketchup, you may prepare and use fresh tomato salsa. Also, instead of using heavy salad dressing, opt to prepare and use vinaigrettes instead, using olive oil, apple cider vinegar, and your choice of herbs.

10.  Refrain from buying dried fruits as these are already loaded with sweeteners and other chemicals such as sulphur dioxide. If you must buy dried fruit, look for those which were sweetened naturally using honey or apple juice.

11. Refrain from buying margarines. Aside from artificial colorings, additives, and emulsifiers to improve appearance, margarines contains chemically hardened vegetable oil. Also, margarines contains trans fat, a type of fat which is not recognized by the body, and hence, may contribute to heart diseases, cancer, bone problems, hormonal imbalance, skin disease, and other health issues. It is better to just use clarified butter, or ghee, than margarine. Clarified butter is butter that has been melted over low hear and allowed to bubble and simmer until most of the water has been evaporated. Butter, despite common misconception about its health benefits, consists of butterfat, as well as some milk

proteins. Butterfat is also known as butyric acid --
the same substance found in a mother's milk.
Other beneficial components of butter include:

a. anti-oxidants such as beta-carotene, selenium, that shield your body from free-radical damage;

b. conjugated linoleic acids, which fights cancer, builds muscle, and boost immunity;

c. iodine, which keeps the thyroid glands healthy;

d. lauric acid, which boosts the immune system and makes it better at fighting infections;

e. lecithin, which has powerful antioxidant properties, and also contributes to cholesterol metabolism, and

f. vitamins A, D, E, and K, which are essential for eye and endocrine health, calcium absorption, healing, skin health, and proper blood clotting.

12. Choose high quality meat. Aim to get
your meat from grass-fed animals as much as
possible. It may be more expensive, but it is a lot
healthier than animals which were fed with feeds
which were also loaded with chemicals from
factories. If you have space and ability, you may
also raise your own chickens. If there is no option

but to purchase lower quality meat, go for the leaner cuts, as chemicals can accumulate in the fatty tissues.

13. Include Healthy Fats. Our body needs fats, so do not be afraid to consume healthy, high-quality saturated fats. Healthy fats is found in fish, such as white tuna, salmon, anchovies and sardines; nuts and seeds such as walnuts, almonds, pecans, chia, flax and hemp seeds; avocados; eggs; and oils such as real butter, olive oil and virgin coconut oil.

14. Consume as many vegetables as you can during your meals. Opt for cruciferous, dark leafy greens. The idea, however, is to have variety of vegetables as possible in your diet, the more colorful, the better.

15. Limit your drink to water. If you must, stick to green tea, coconut water, and aloe vera juice. Moderate the intake of coffee.

16. For purposes of weight loss, you may want to stock up on these foods:

a. Whole eggs. Eggs are high in protein, healthy fats, and can make you feel full with a very low amount of calories. In a study of overweight women, it was showed that eating eggs for breakfast increased satiety and caused the women to eat less for the next thirty-six (36) hours.

b. Leafy greens and cruciferous vegetables. Leafy greens and cruciferous vegetables are loaded with fiber while containing low carbohydrates. Eating leafy greens and cruciferous vegetables during meals can help you consume less calories while getting enough nutrients and satiety. The fiber in the food will also help regulate bowel movement. Cruciferous vegetables includes broccoli, cauliflower, cabbage, garden cress, and brussels sprouts.

c. Seafood. Seafood contains iodine, which is necessary for the proper function of the thyroid, which regulates metabolism.

d. Lean Beef and Chicken Breast. Unprocessed lean beef and chicken breast contains a lot of protein, which is the most fulfilling nutrient. Eating a high-protein diet can make you burn up to a hundred more calories per day.

e.  Beans and Legumes. Beans and legumes are high in protein and fiber, which will help a person feel full. Beans and legumes also contain resistant starch, which allows for sustained energy release.

f.  Cottage Cheese. Cheese in general is high in protein. However, cottage cheese has the highest amount of protein, and very little carbohydrate and fat.

g.  Avocados. Avocados are loaded with healthy fats and high in monounsaturated oleic acid, which is the same fat found in olive oil. Avocados are perfect additions to salads, as studies have shown that fats in avocados increases the nutrient uptake from the vegetables.

h.  Apple Cider Vinegar (ACV). Taking ACV at the same time as a high carbohydrate meal can increase the feeling of fullness and can make a person eat less calories throughout the day. ACV can also aid digestion and regulate bowel movement.

i.   Grapefruit. Studies have shown that people who eat grapefruit before meals where able to lose weight. Moreover, grapefruit can help people suffering from insulin resistance and metabolic abnormality.

j.   Chia Seeds. Chia seeds is one of the best source of fiber known to man. Because of its fiber content, these seeds can absorb up to 11-12 times of their weight in water, expands in the stomach, and makes a person feel full.

You may try this five (5) day meal plan which applies the above principles to get you started!

Day 1:

---

**Breakfast - Wholegrain cereal with milk, topped with ½ cup blue berries and 200 g. low fat fruit yogurt.**

---

Lunch – Tuna salad roll

You will need:

1 Wholemeal roll, sliced avocadoes, chopped tune (cooked), cheese, carrot strips, 2 slices of beetroot, and cucumber slices.

Dinner- Baked lean turkey breast with vegetables

You will need:

200g Turkey breast, glazed in honey or marinated in sauce, steamed squash and broccoli as sides.

Snacks - Whole-wheat bread topped with cottage cheese and fresh tomato, green tea.

Day 2:

Breakfast – 1 toasted whole meal flat bread topped with cheese. 1 banana and 20g wholegrain cereal with skimmed milk.

Lunch – Wholemeal beef bread roll

You will need:

1 wholemeal, 60g Lean roast beef, avocado slices, 2 tsp honey, grated carrots, chopped cucumber, and lettuce

Dinner

Marinated chicken skewers and chickpea salad

You will need:

200 g Chicken breast marinated in 1 tsp olive oil, cumin, fresh garlic, coriander, and mint

¾ cup Chick pea,  ½ cup English spinach, ¼ cup cherry tomatoes, 3 onion rings, 1 tsb parsley, and citrus dressing,

Snacks

1 apple, diced and mixed with low-fat yogurt, green tea.

Day 3:

---

Breakfast – Mixed fruits (we recommend: apples, pears, bananas, and oranges – or any combination thereof) topped with about 200g of vanilla yogurt and 20g whole grain cereal.

Lunch – Wholemeal tuna bread roll

You will need:

1 wholemeal, 60g tuna, 2 tsp honey, grated carrots, chopped cucumber, tettuce

---

| Dinner |
| --- |
| Vegetable soup and garlic prawns |
| You will need: |
| Cauliflower, beans, broccoli, carrots |
| Sauteed garlic and prawns |
| 1 heavily seeded bread roll and butter |

| Snacks |
| --- |
| Two soy linseed corn crispbreads and green tea. Optional: top bread with cheese. |

Day 4:

| Breakfast – 40g cereal, wholegrain, topped with 200g vanilla yogurt, a tablespoon of chia seeds, 3 prunes and 3 apricot halves (dried) |
| --- |

Lunch – Crispbread topped with eggs and tuna

You will need:

4 crispbread, egg, tuna

1 apple

---

Dinner

Creamy chicken pasta

You will need:

200g skinless chicken breast, ¼ cup light evaporated milk, chicken stock, 4 asparagus spears, ¼ cup frozen peas and corn, 1 cup cooked wholemeal pasta

---

Snacks

Fruit slices of your choice

Day 5:

---

Breakfast – apple and banana smoothie, with 40g wholegrain cereal with skim milk

Lunch – Sardines on toast

You will need:

2 slices wholemeal toast, butter, and sardines in tomato sauce

1 cup of green grapes

Dinner

Beef and spinach pasta and salad

You will need:

200g lean beef,     ½ cup English spinach, ¼ cup light evaporated milk, tomato puree,  fress garlic and basil, 1 cup cooked wholemeal pasta

½ cup lettuce, ¼ cup mushrooms, sliced cucumber, 5 olives, 1 tsp olive oil, ½ tsp balsamic vinegar, and ½ tsp honey, wholegrain mustard

Snacks

Mixed apple, banana, and orange, topped with light cream.

Keep in mind that the following are mere guidelines to help you in achieving a healthier lifestyle, as there is no one-size-fits-all definition of clean eating. The general rule is to eat wholesome foods, and avoid chemically laden food. Keep in mind that each individual has a different genetic make-up, and hence, our dietary needs are different. Also clean eating is not merely a phase, or a diet that you can do for a week, or a month, in order for you to lose weight. Your decision to live healthy and eat clean, wholesome foods must be a lifestyle change, which ultimately redefines your relationship with food. Otherwise, the exercise will be futile.

Moreover, keep in mind that clean eating is not equivalent to self-deprivation. Sure, you may be taking in fewer calories than before, but it does not mean that you will starve yourself. As a matter of fact, eating clean can allow you to eat more. You might be surprise to know that a quarter bar of your favorite white chocolate has the same calorie content as a big bowl of greens! Also, eating lean proteins such as chicken breast, fish, tofu, and green such as broccoli, kale, lettuce, green beans, together with whole grains like quinoa, oatmeal, and brown rice can keep you feel fuller for a longer time.

Keep in mind also that the goal of clean eating is not to frustrate the individual, but to keep him or her happy and healthy. Hence, if you really want to try that piece of cake in a party, do it, but do not over do it. The idea is to live healthy most of the time, not to have a perfect tract record., below is the comparison by NYC Health between the current serving size and the serving size during the 1980's:

| Food | 1980s | Present |
|------|-------|---------|
| Turkey sandwich | 320 calories | 820 calories |
| French fries | 210 calories | 610 calories |

| | | |
|---|---|---|
| Bagel | 140 calories | 350 calories |
| Slice of Pizza | 500 calories | 850 calories |
| Soda | 85 calories | 250 calories |

Hence, in order to properly lead a clean eating lifestyle, you must be conscious of the portions of the food you eat. For example, even though real butter is healthy for you, it is not advisable to put cups of butter to your food. Food portion can be easily controlled using your hands as guide, as follows:

| Food | Portion | Equivalent serving size |
|---|---|---|
| Cheese | One pointer finger | 1 and ½ ounces |
| Milk and yogurt | One fist | 1 cup |

| | | |
|---|---|---|
| Cooked carrots (or others of similar appearance) | One fist | 1 cup |
| Salad | Two fists | 2 cups |
| Fruits | One fist | 1 cup |
| Dry cereal | One fist | 1 cup |
| Noodles, rice, oatmeal | A handful | ½ cup |

| Slice of whole wheat bread | Flat Hand | 1 slice |
|---|---|---|
| Chicken, beef, fish, pork | Palm | 3 ounces |
| Butter, peanut butter, jams, dressings | Thumb | 1 tablespoon |

Source: Dairy Council of California

Reading food labels, and paying attention to the number of servings stated in the labels is also a great way to avoid over-estimating your portions. It will also be wise to re-packed big bags of food to ample serving sizes.

# 5 GOOD MOOD FOOD

Aside from fueling your body, the right type of food can be a good way to boost your mood and energy. Stock on the following food to ward away slump days:

1. Bananas. Bananas are some of the best foods that you can munch on to supply your body with energy. Bananas are rich in potassium and B vitamins, and can provide your body with more sustained released of energy. Moreover, bananas make you feel full and keep blood sugar levers stable.

2. Salmon. Salmon is a great source of energy-boosting omega-3 fatty acids, which are essential for energy production, brain activity and circulation.

3. Coconut. The oils in coconuts consists of a medium chain triglycerides, a type of fat that is turned into energy quickly and efficiently. Also, the body utilizes coconut to produce energy rather than store it as fat.

4. Lentils and legumes. Lentils and legumes help stabilize blood glucose levels and prevent mid-afternoon slumps.

5. Eggs. Eggs are good sources of iron and protein. They are also naturally rich in B-Vitamins which are responsible for converting food into energy.

6. Kale. Kale is considered by many as a superfood. It is high in vitamins and minerals such as copper, potassium, iron and phosphorous which essential for an energy-boost.

7. Ginger Tea. Instead of taking coffee, why not try ginger tea instead? Ginger tea is filled with anti-oxidants and nutrients to provide your body with sustained energy throughout the day.

8. Nuts. Nuts such as almonds, cashews, and hazelnuts, are all high in magnesium,

which is essential for the conversion of sugar into energy. They are also filled with fiber which keep your blood sugar levels in check.

9. Quinoa. Quinoa is a gluten-free grain that contains more protein than any other grain or rice. It is also rich in amino acids that is considered as a complete protein source. It is high in lysine, methionine, and cysteine, folate, magnesium, phosphorous, and manganese.

10. Goji Berries. Goji berries has been used for thousands of years to help increase energy and enhance the released of hormones. Goji berries also enhances our bodies ability to handle stress, supports healthy mood, mind and memory.

11. Asparagus. Asparagus is one of the best plant-based sources of tryptophan which helps create serotonin, which is the brain's primary mood-regulating neurotransmitters. Asparagus also has a high level of folate to add to its mood-boosting effects.

12. Raw Cacao. Good news for the chocolate lovers! Nibbling on a square or two of dark chocolate (not below 70%) can

energize your body by providing excellent source of iron and magnesium.

# CONCLUSION

I want to thank you again for downloading this book!

I sincerely hope through reading this, you are able to acquire the happiness and health you've always wanted and can rid yourself of that unwanted weight and gain more energy to be as productive as possible throughout your day.

The next step is to put the knowledge you have learned into action!

### **Stay Happy & Stay Healthy**

Finally, if you enjoyed this book, I would be more than appreciative if you would take not even two minutes to leave a review on Amazon.

Blessings to you and good luck!

Also, check out alkalineartists.com to get your hands on a sample of the purest alkaline water available to benefit your health (Alkaline Artists - Kangen Water).

# ABOUT THE AUTHOR

L.T. Currow is a fresh-faced non-fiction writer covering a variety of topics. Mr. Currow enjoys reading fiction and non-fiction books of numerous genres. His hobbies include sailing and venturing on wine tastings. A travel aficionado, Currow resides in sunny San Diego, CA with his two beautiful greyhounds, Meryl and Horace.